THIS NOTEBOOK BELONGS TO

DEAR COLORING LOVER,

THANK YOU SO MUCH FOR PURSHASING OUR BOOK! OUR TEAM WORKED HARD WITH HEART TO MAKE SUCH A WONDERFUL BOOK FOR YOU.

WE GENUINELY HOPE YOU ENJOY THIS SNARCKY COLORING BOOK.

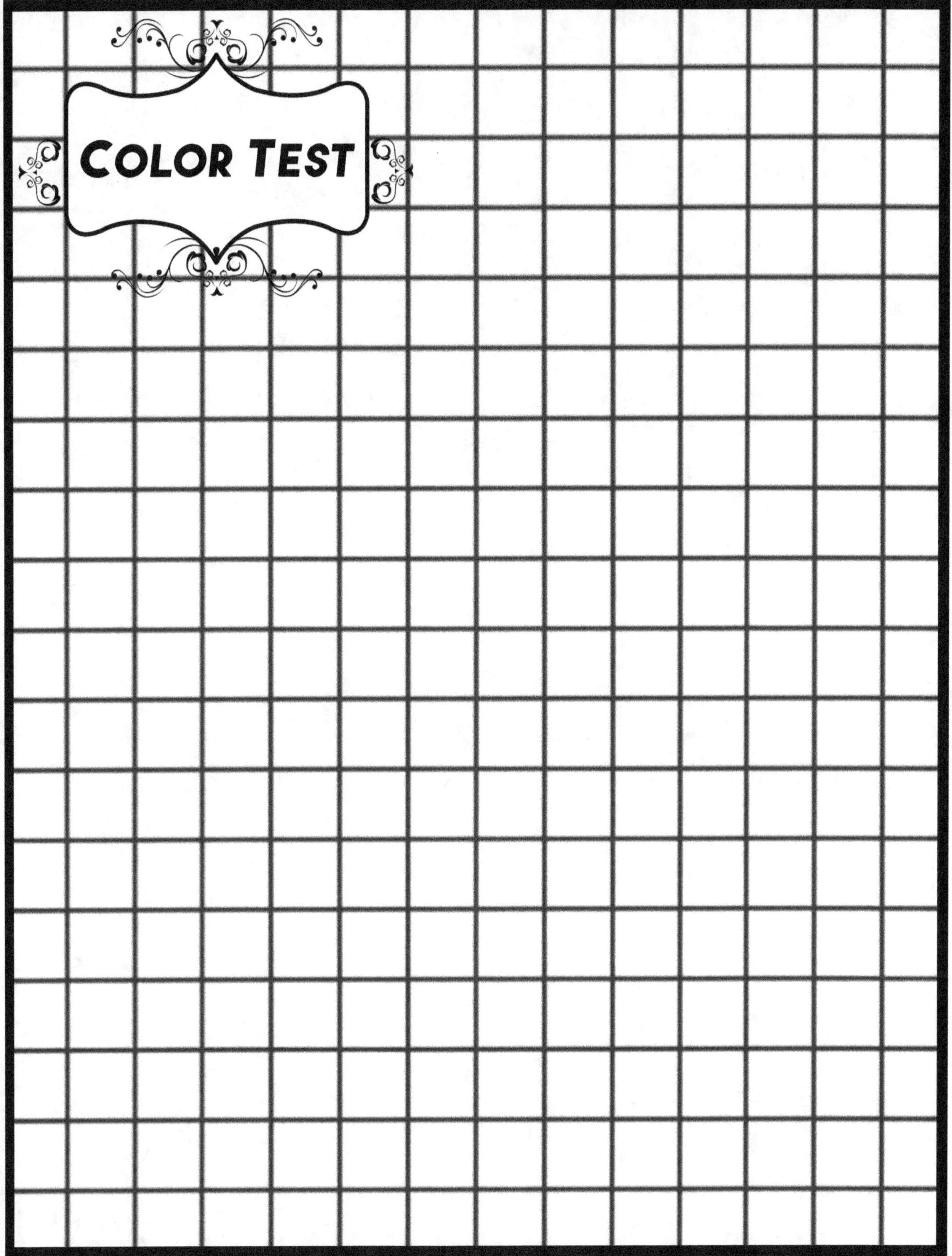
COLOR TEST

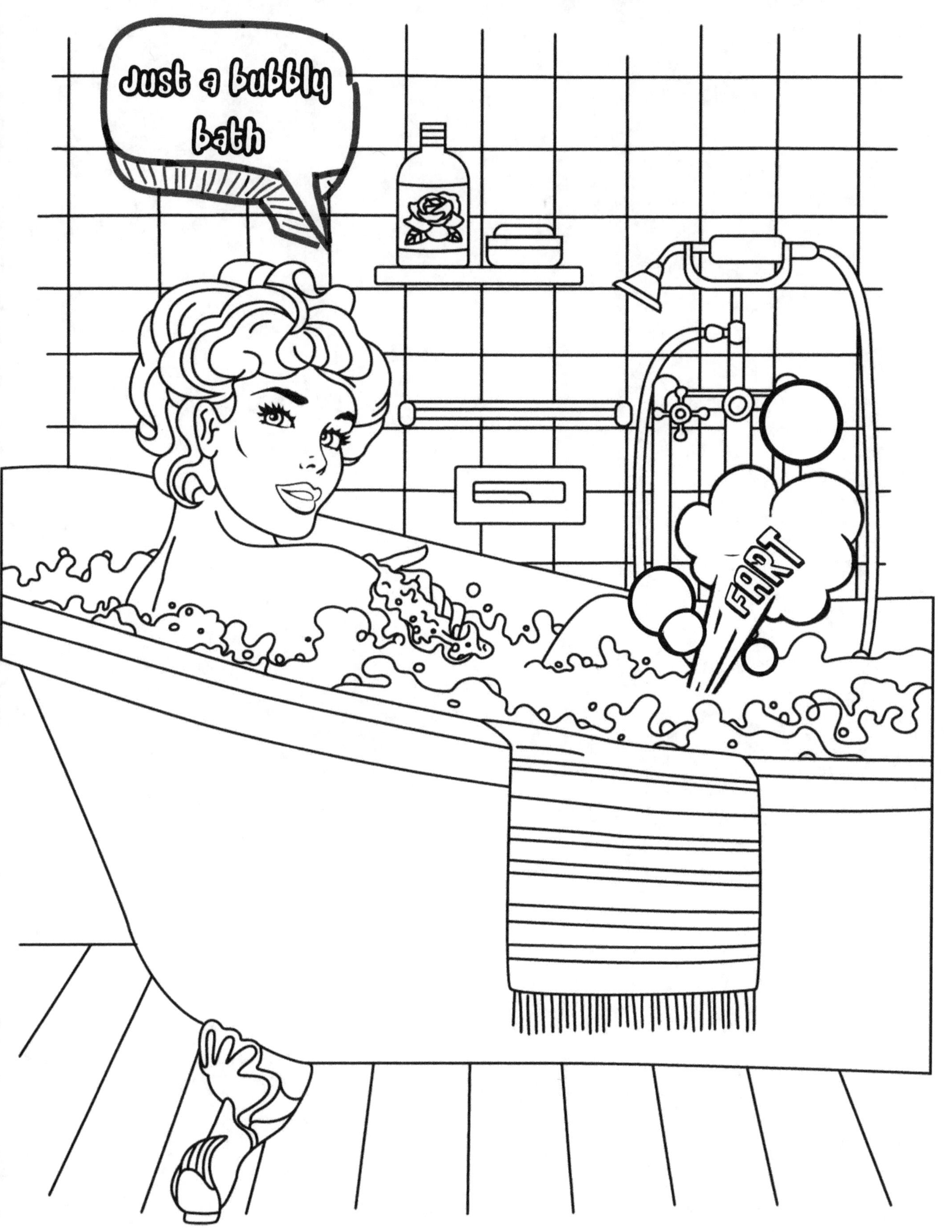

Just a bubbly bath
FART

Mmm what a smell

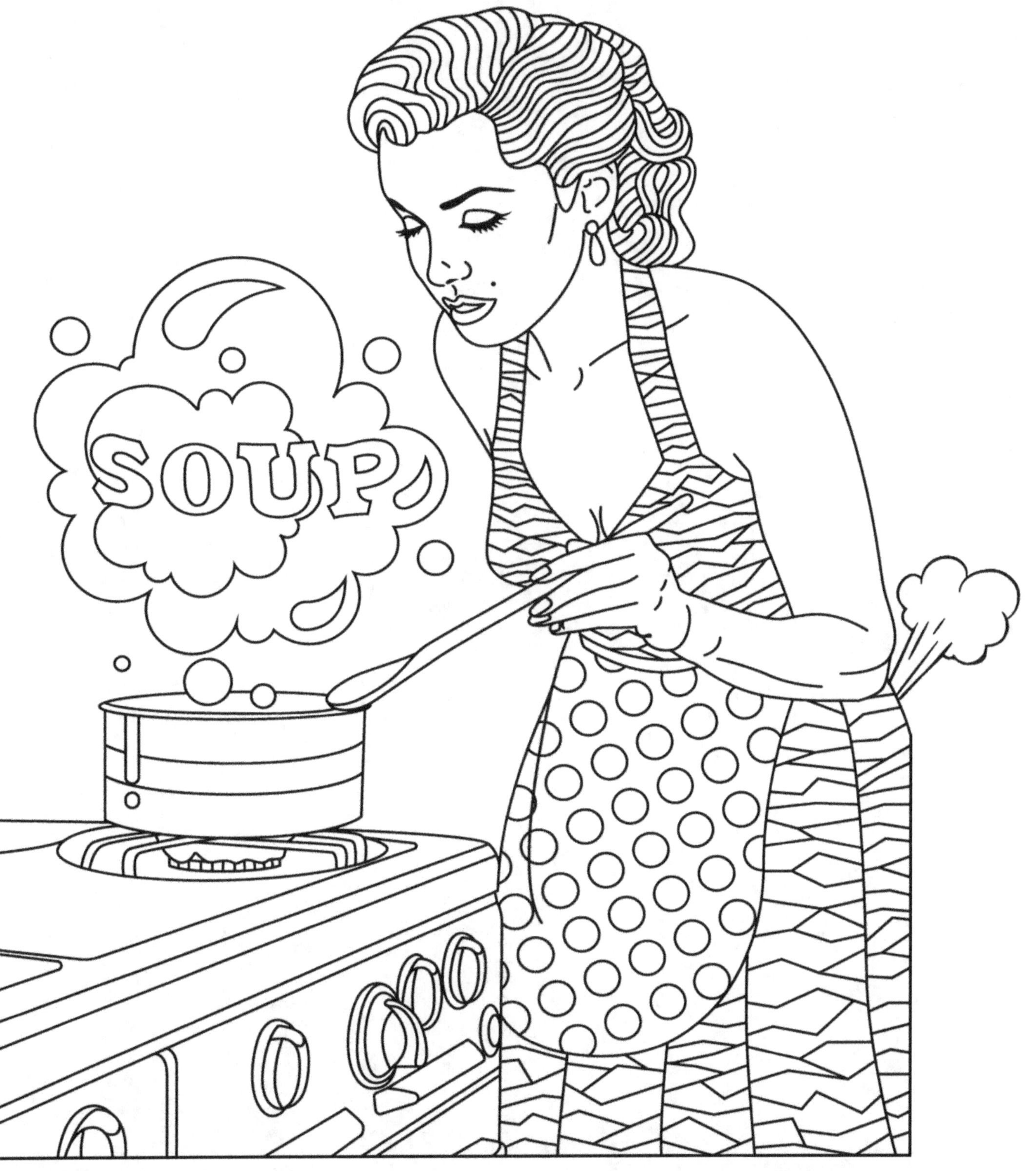

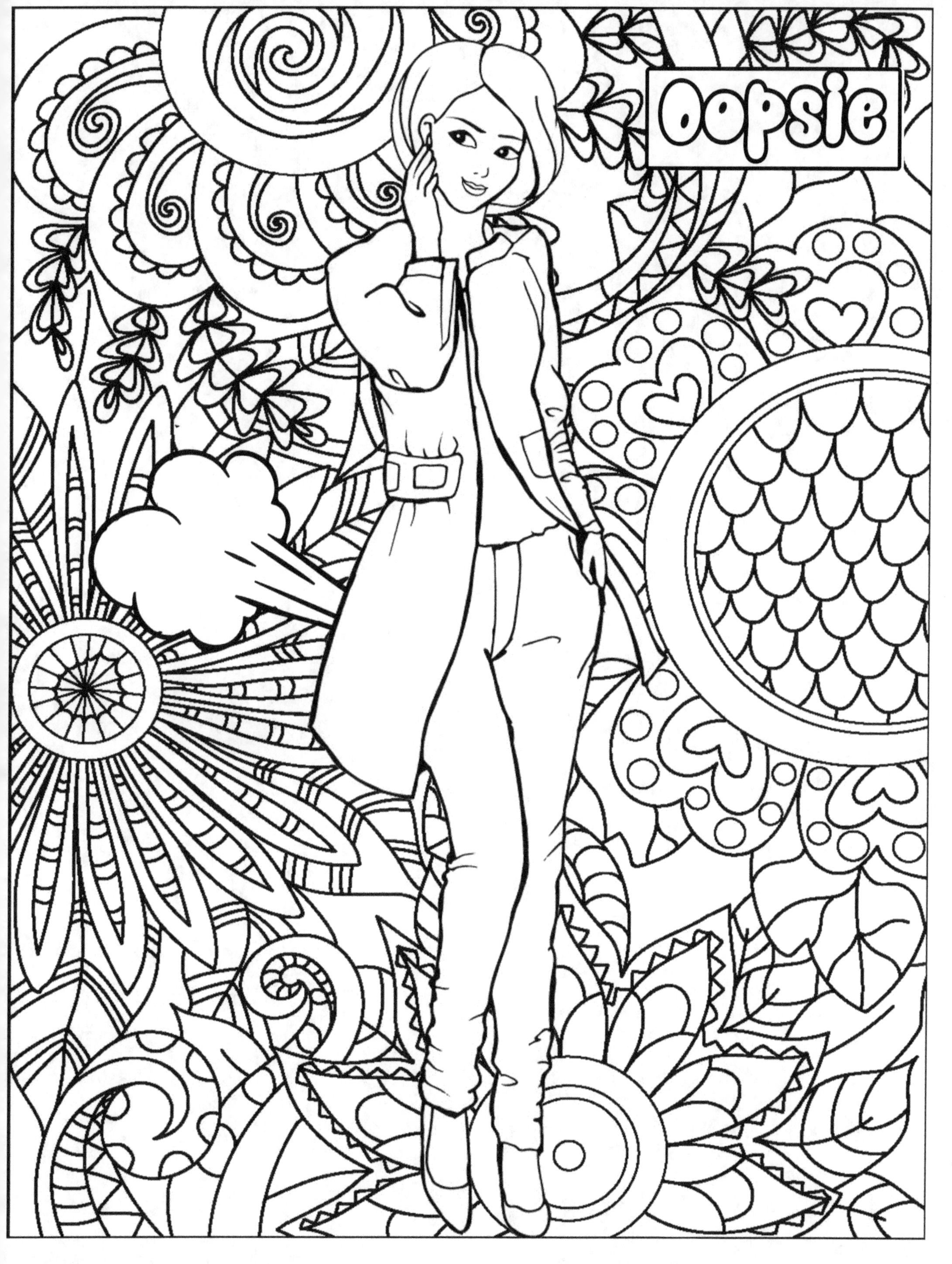

Oopsie

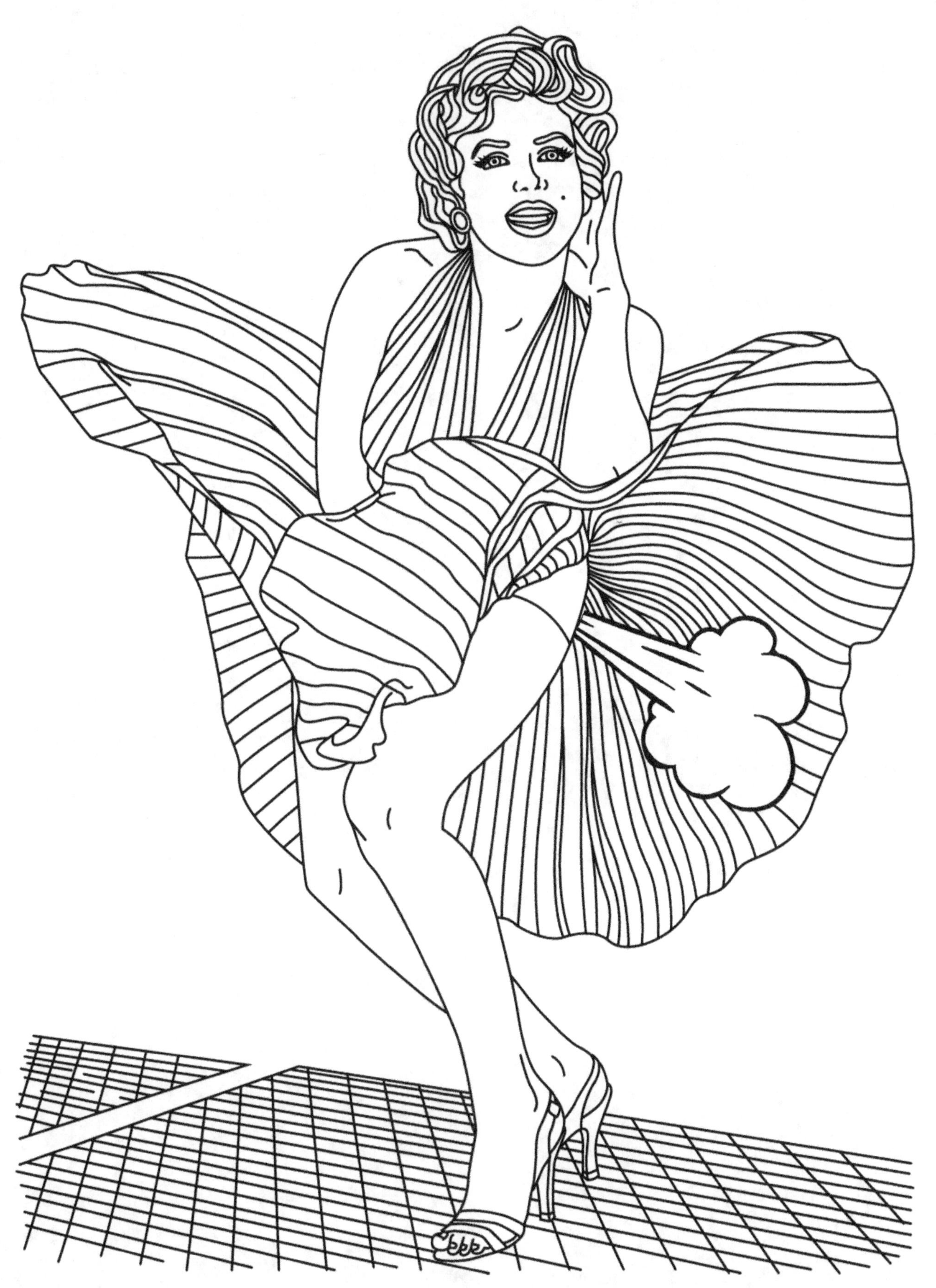

Not me..

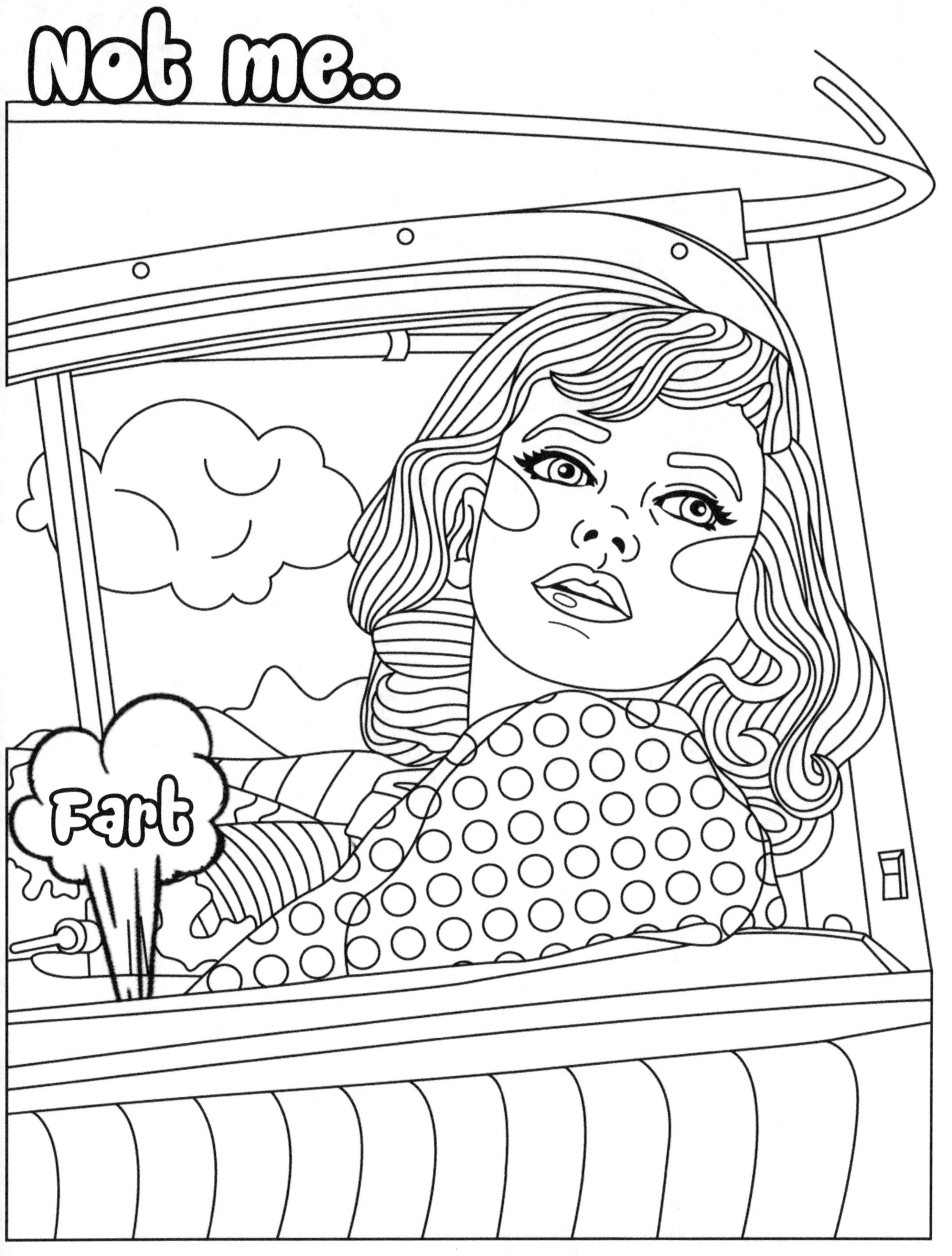

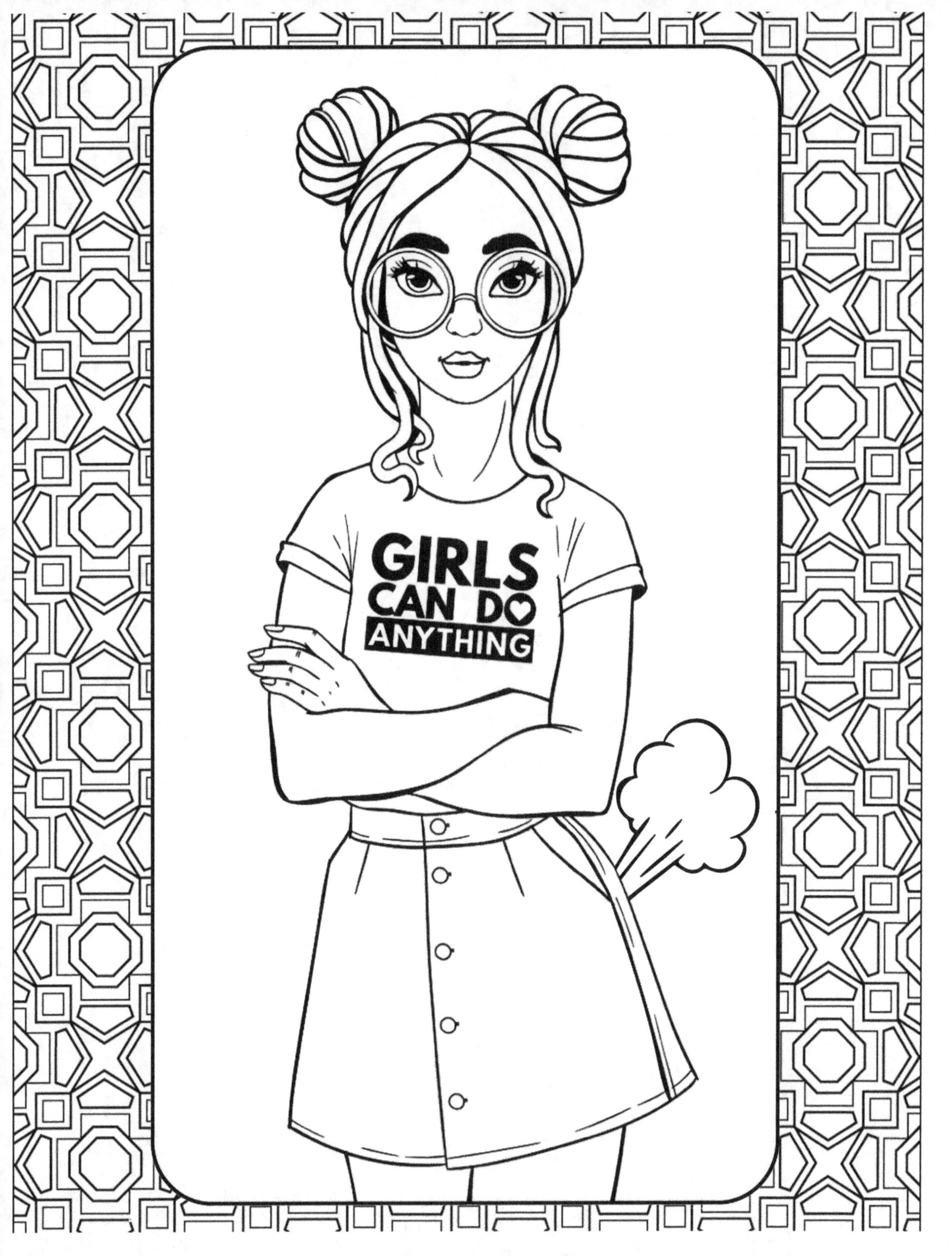

GIRLS
CAN DO
ANYTHING

Feels Good Man

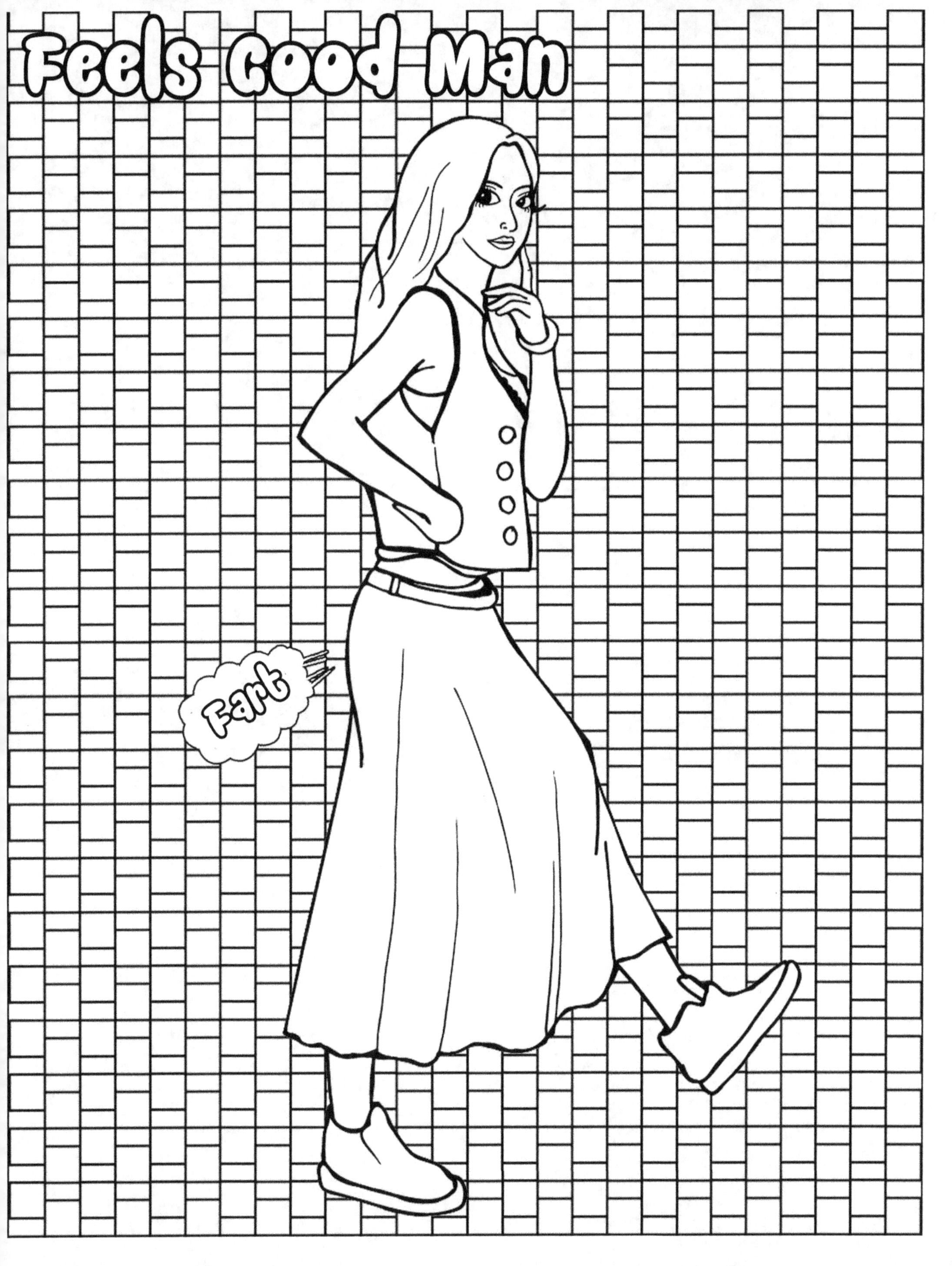

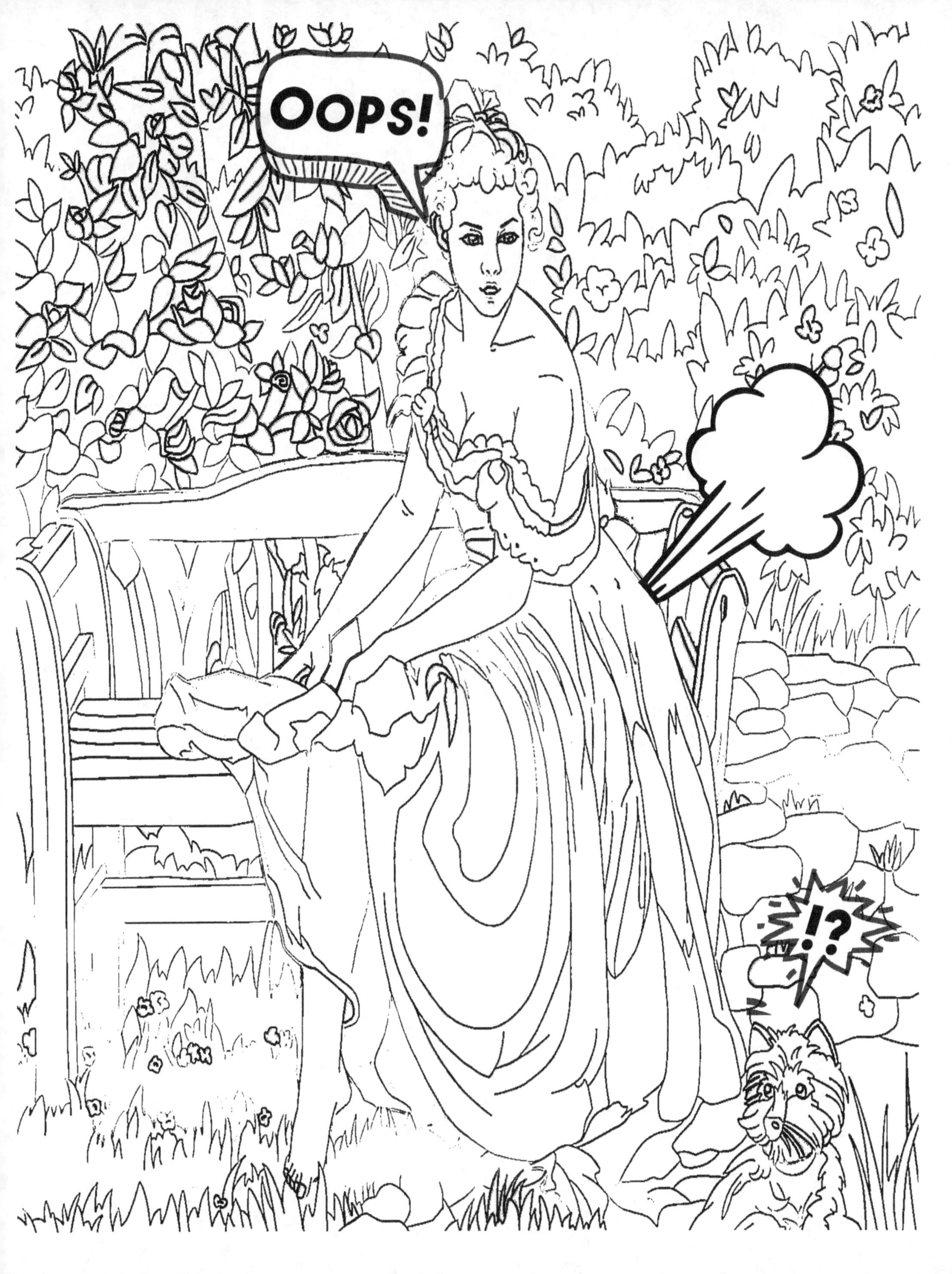

OOPS!
!?

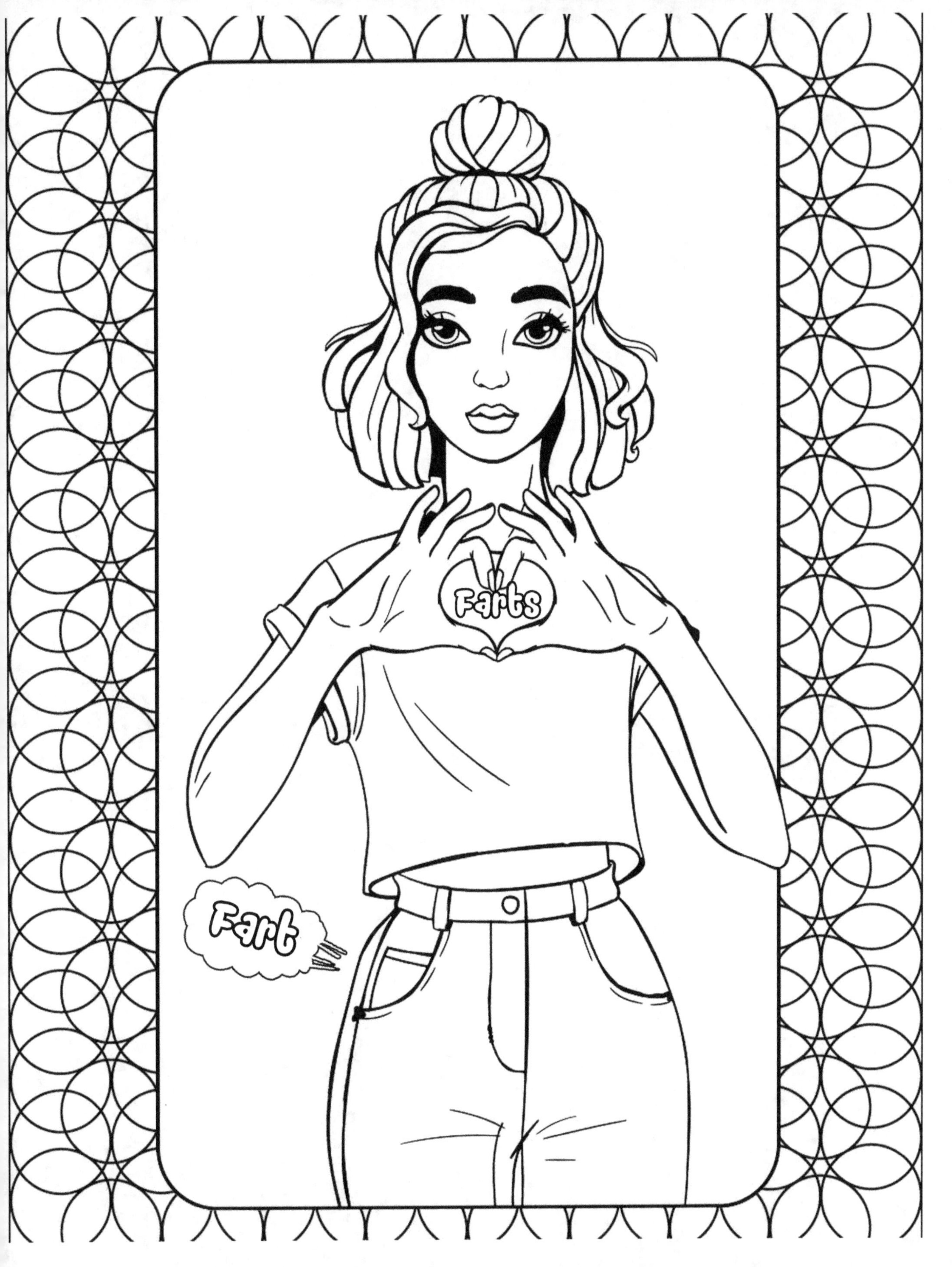
Farts
Fart

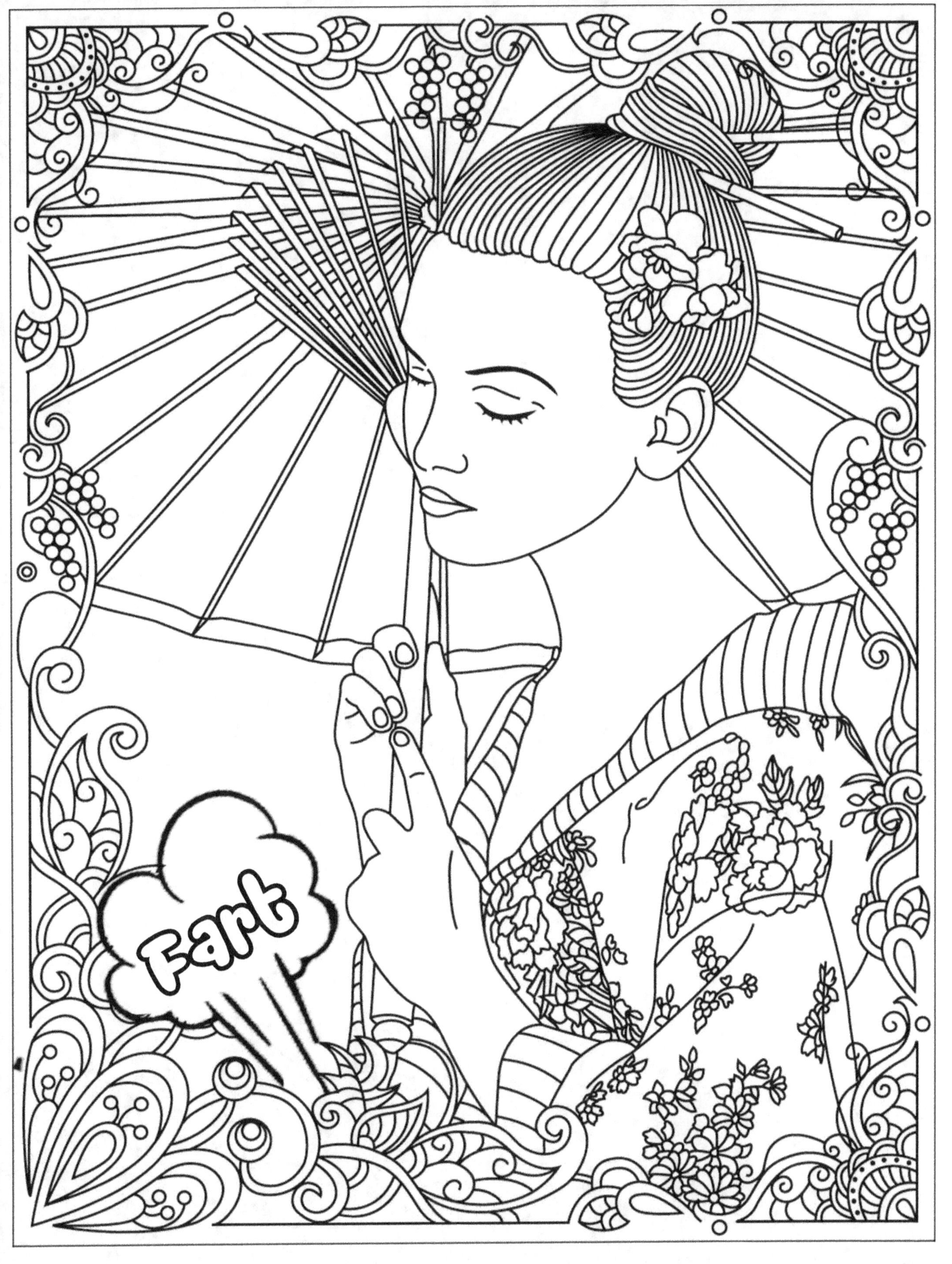
Fart

I don't Always Fart But When I do I don't

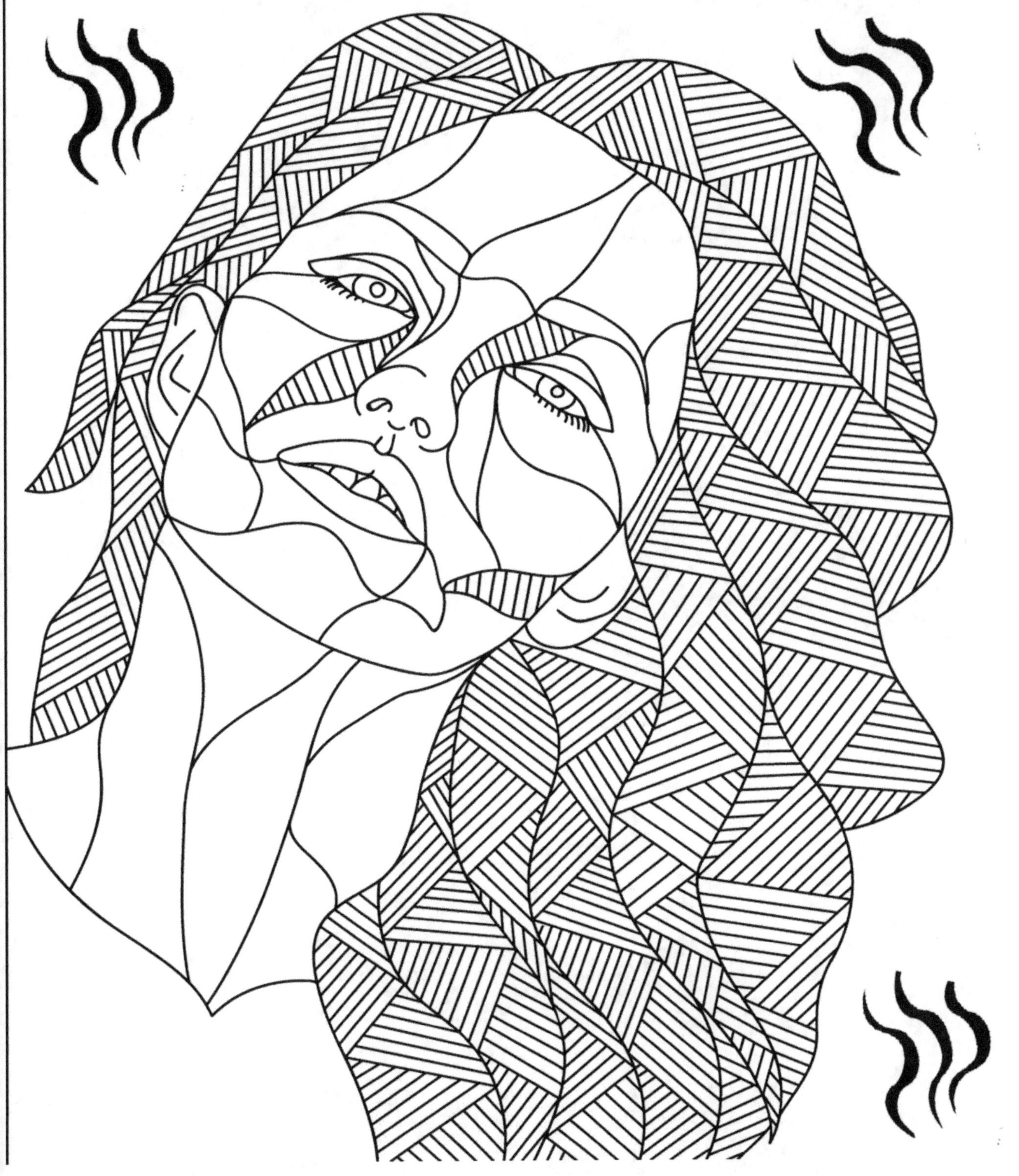

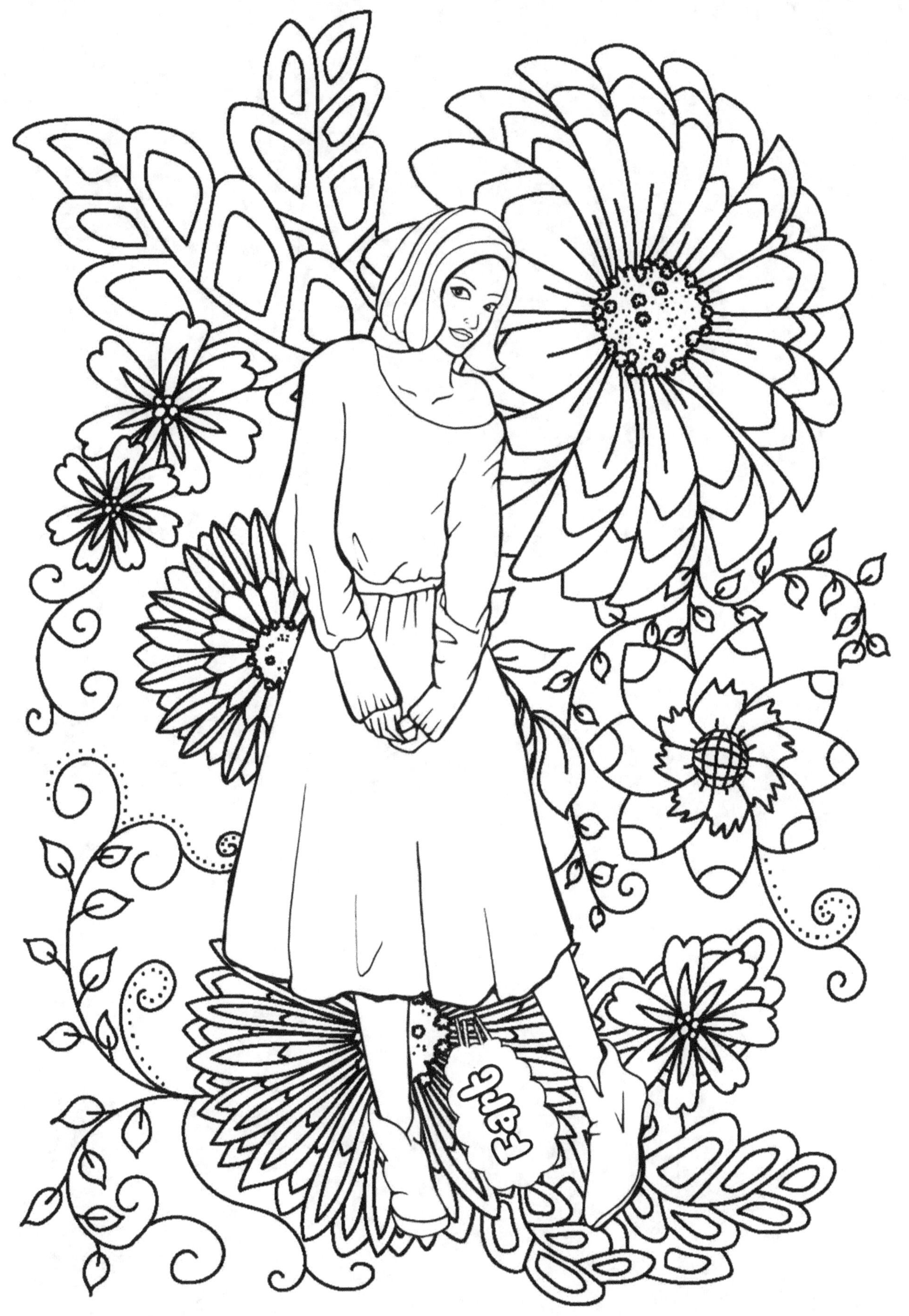
Faith

My bad...

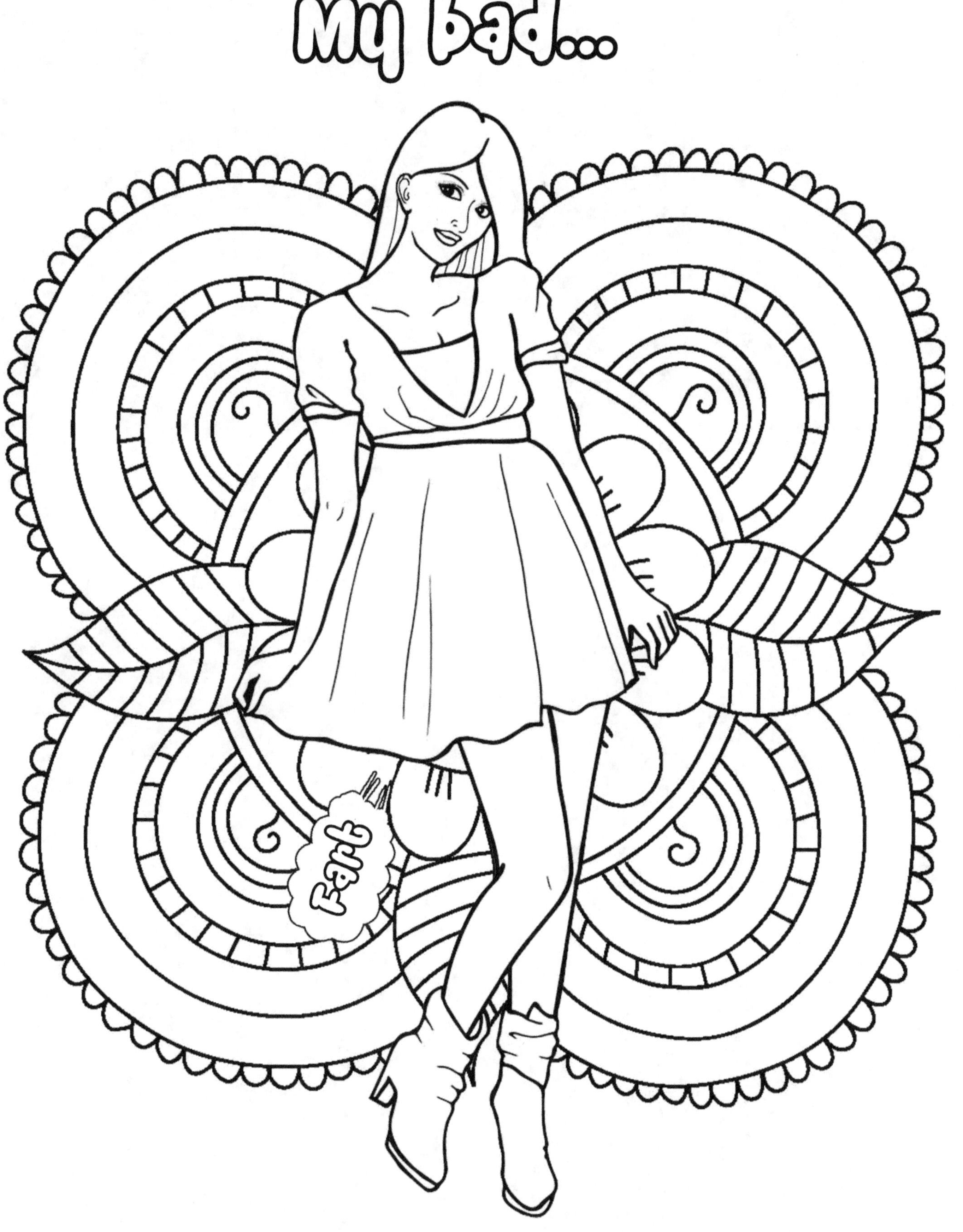

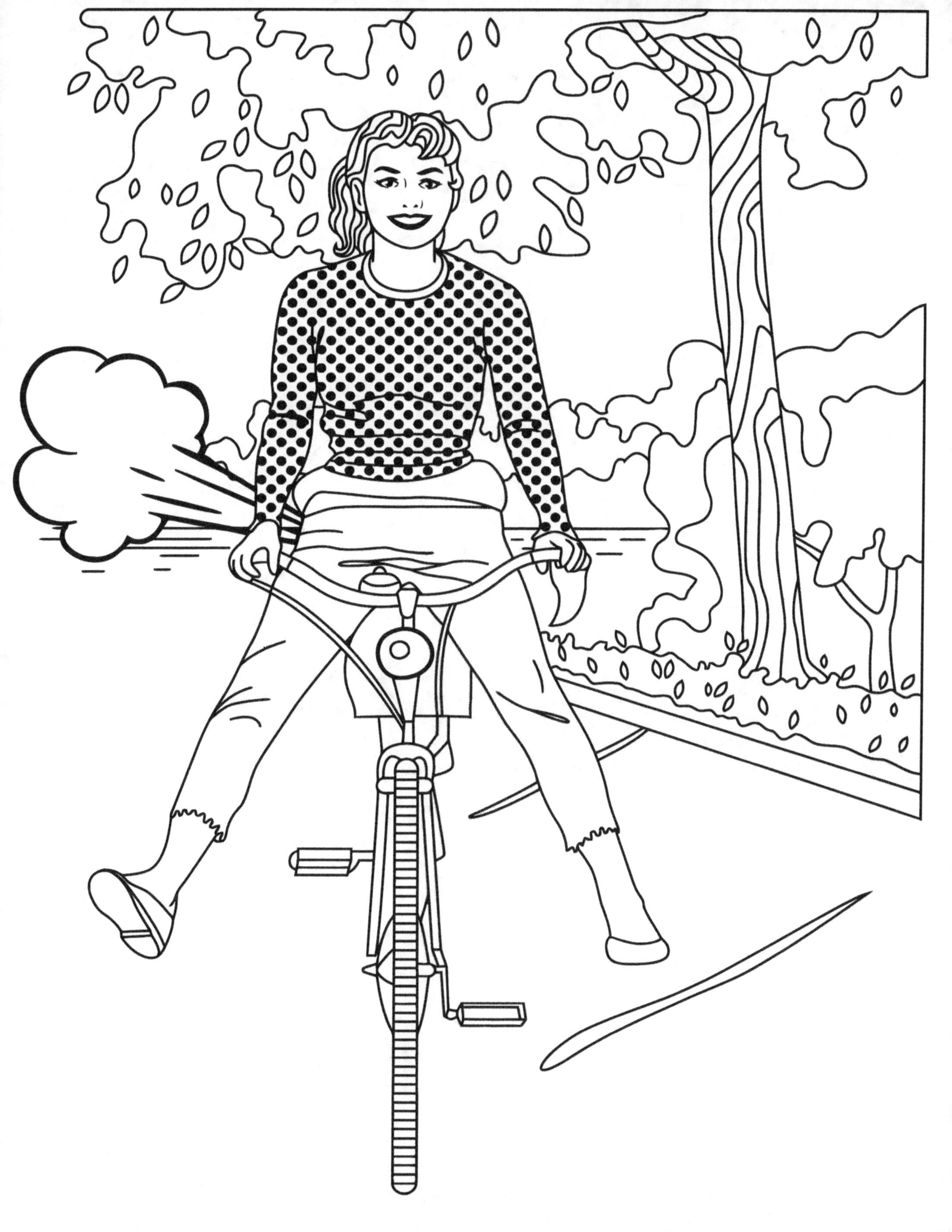

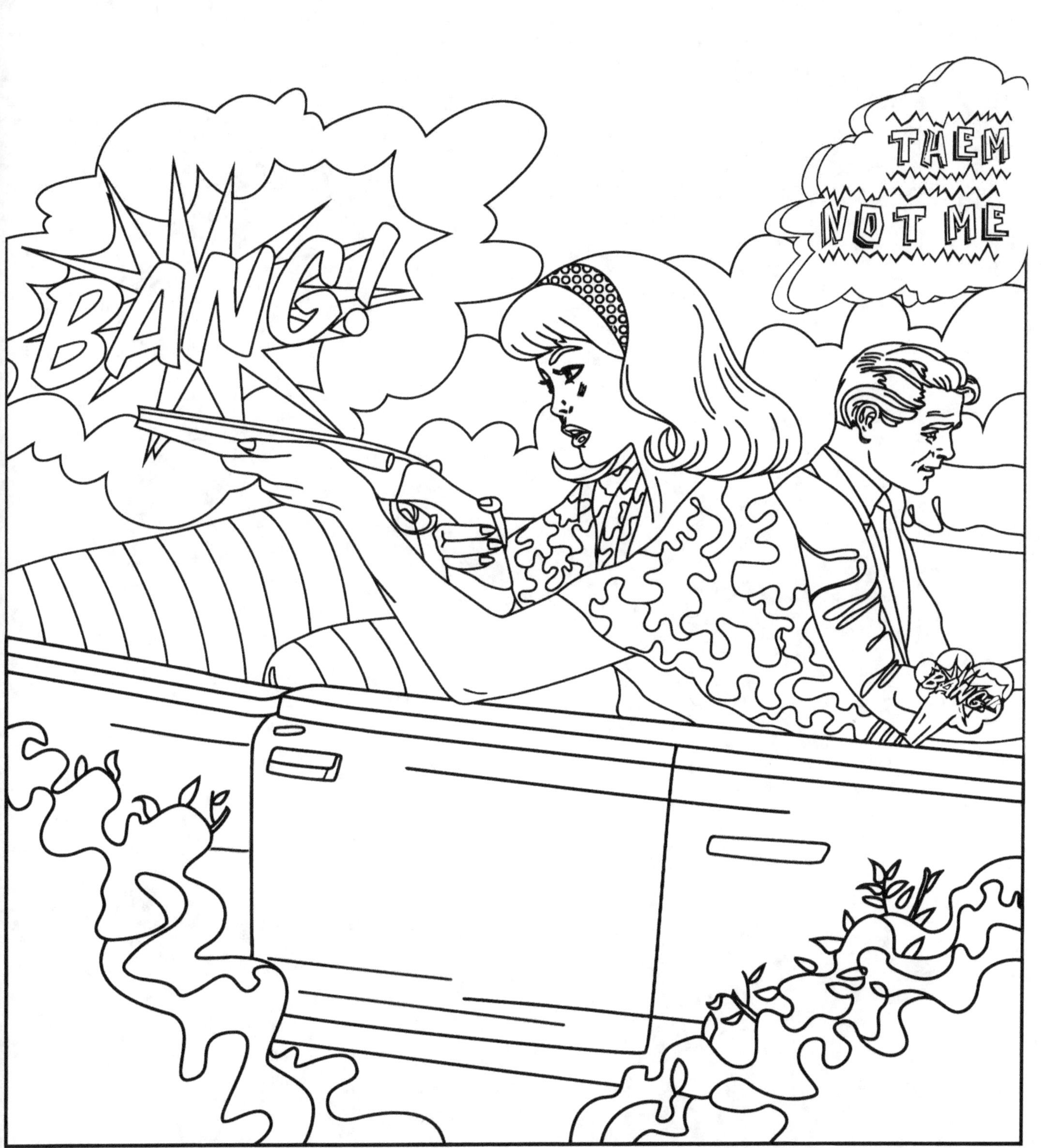

BANG!
THEM NOT ME
BANG

OOPS

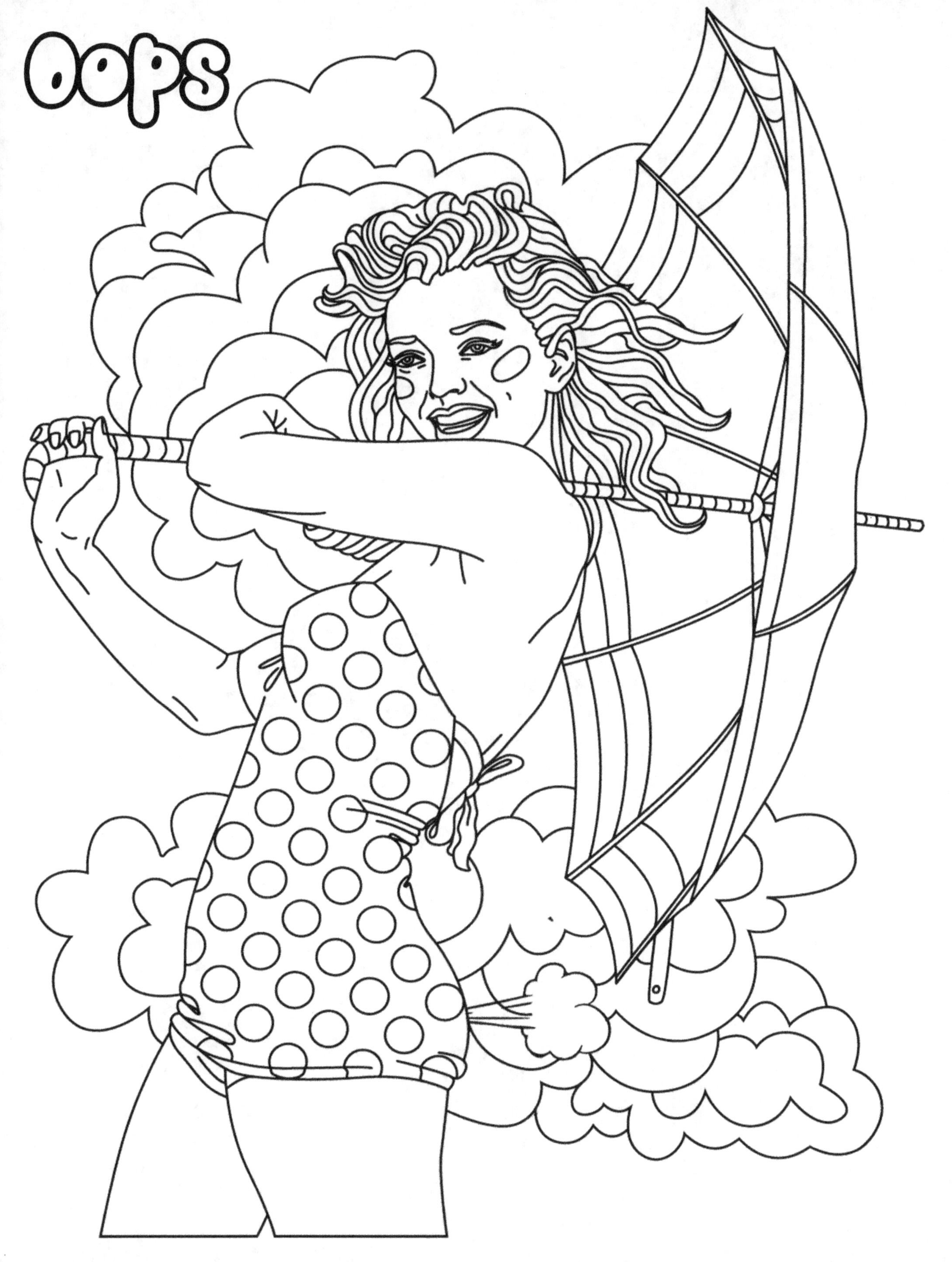

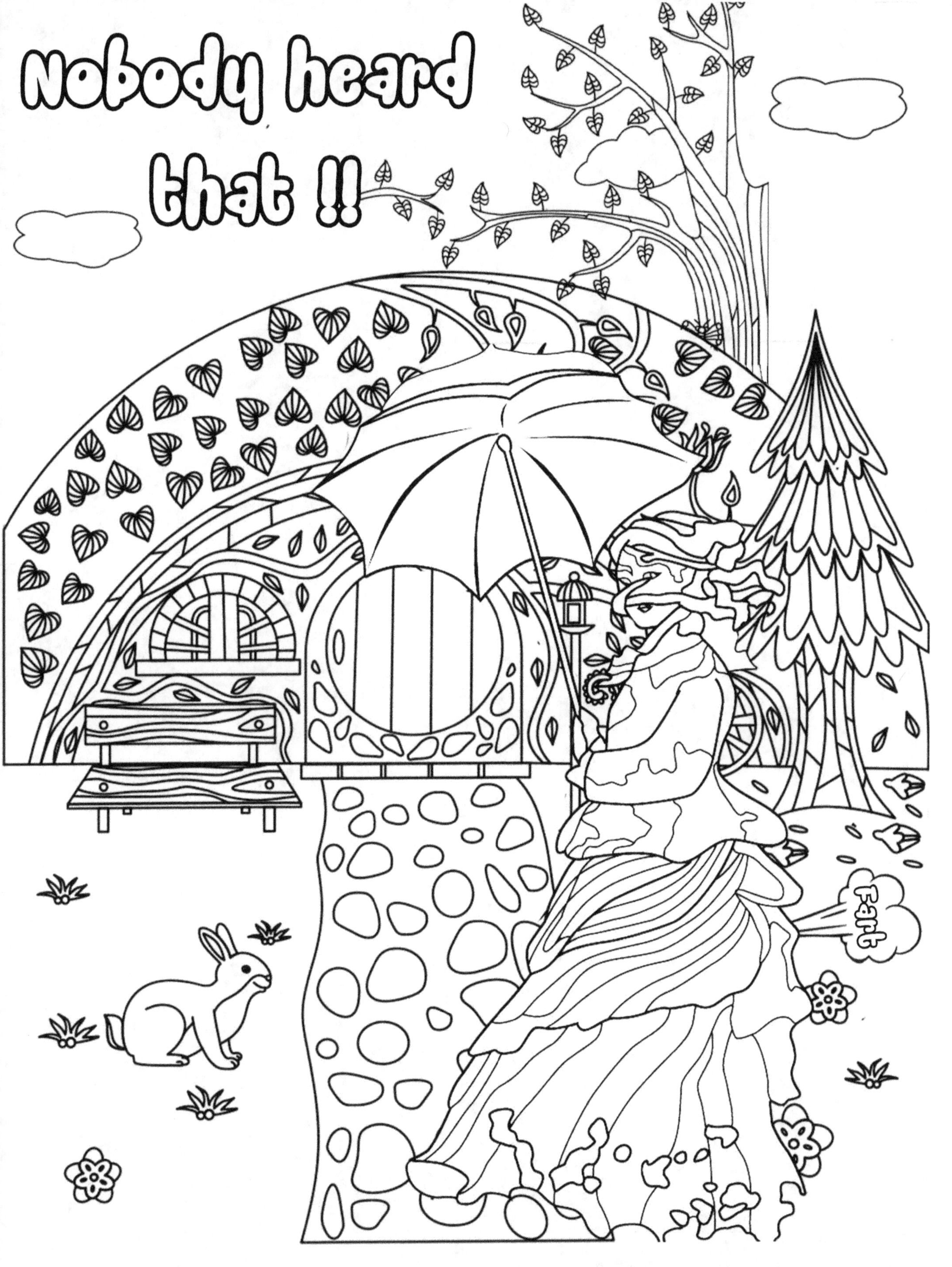

Nobody heard
that !!
Fart

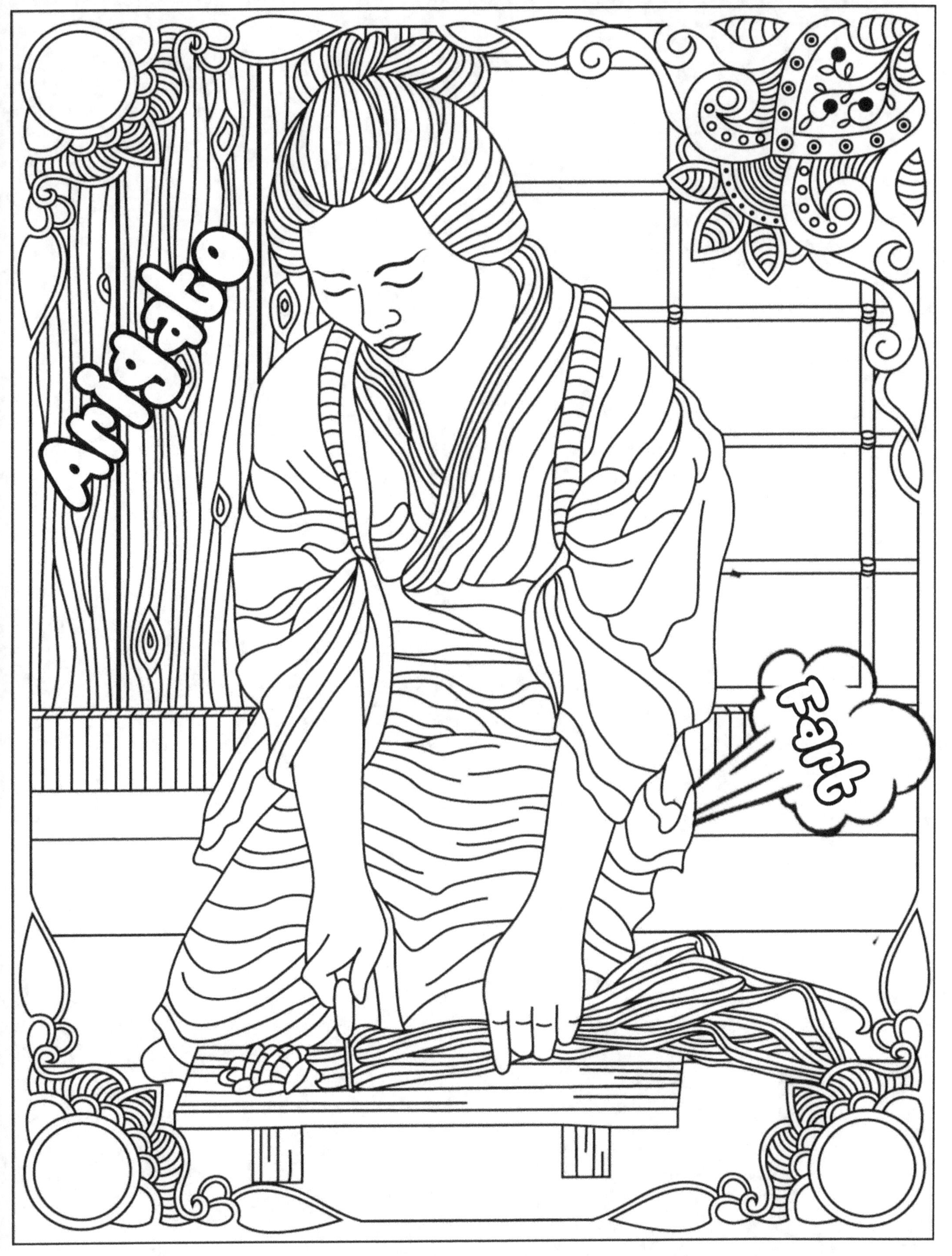
Arigato
Fart

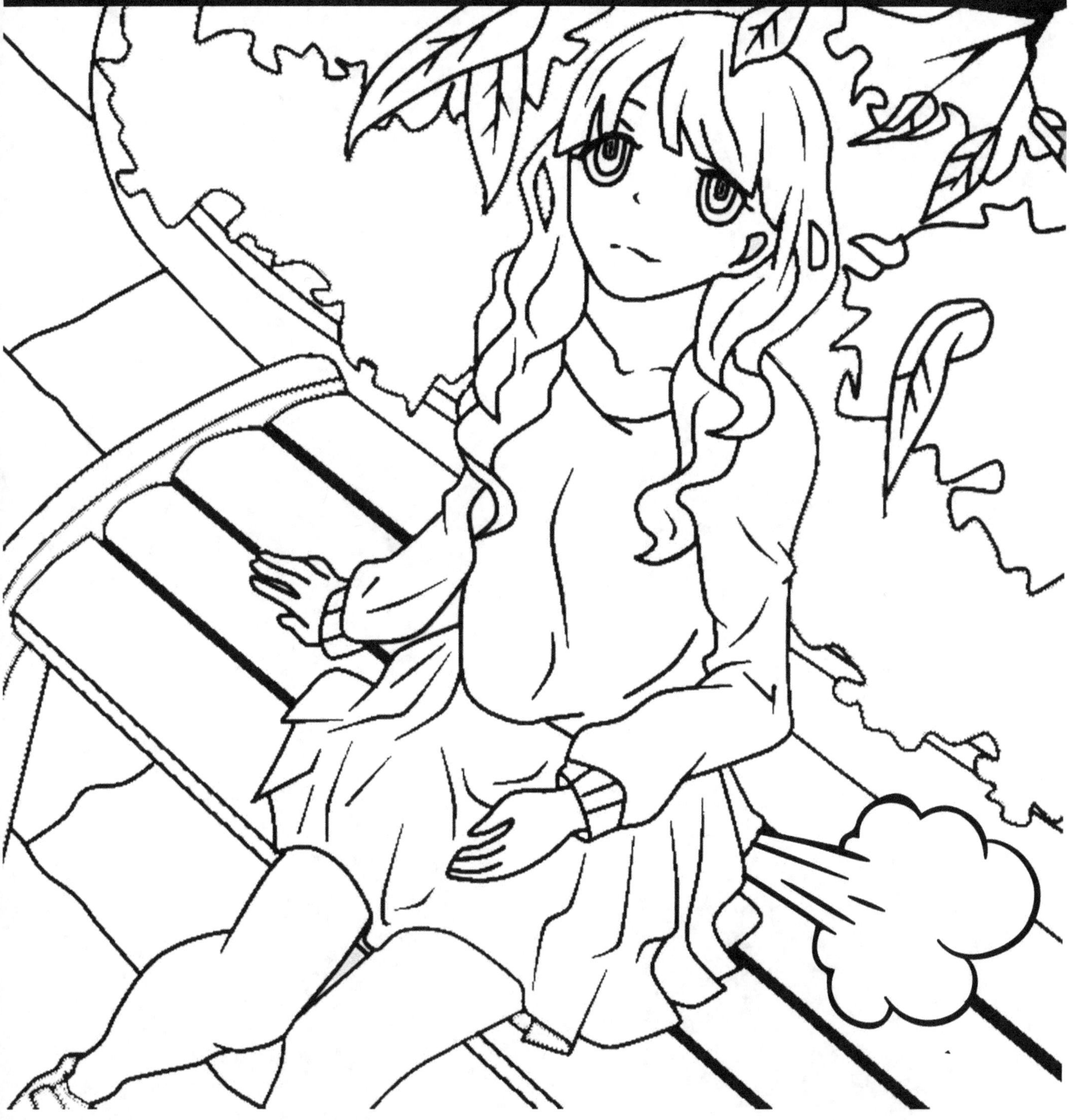
Finally..

what are you looking at

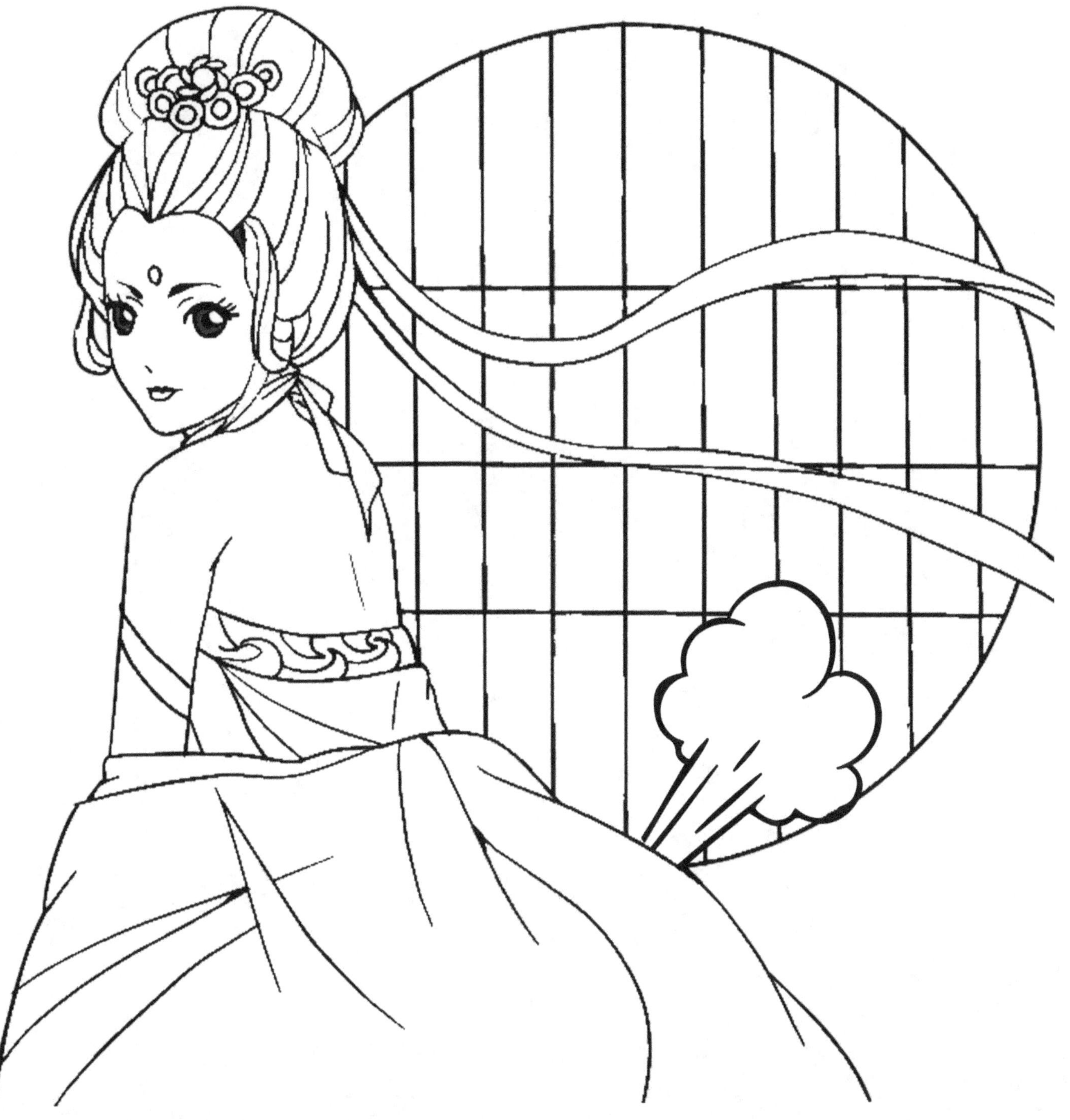

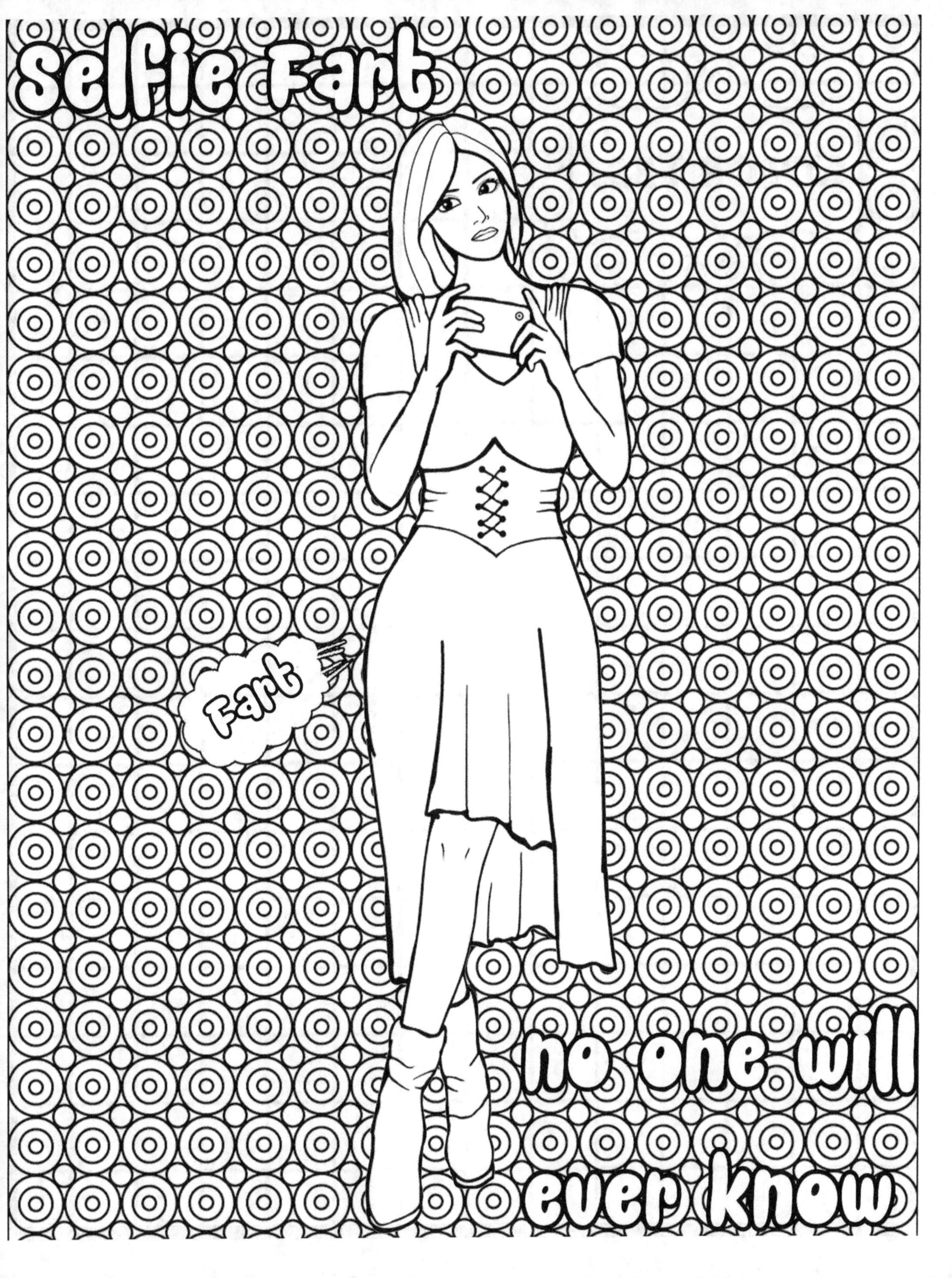
Selfie Fart
Fart
no one will ever know

COLOR TEST

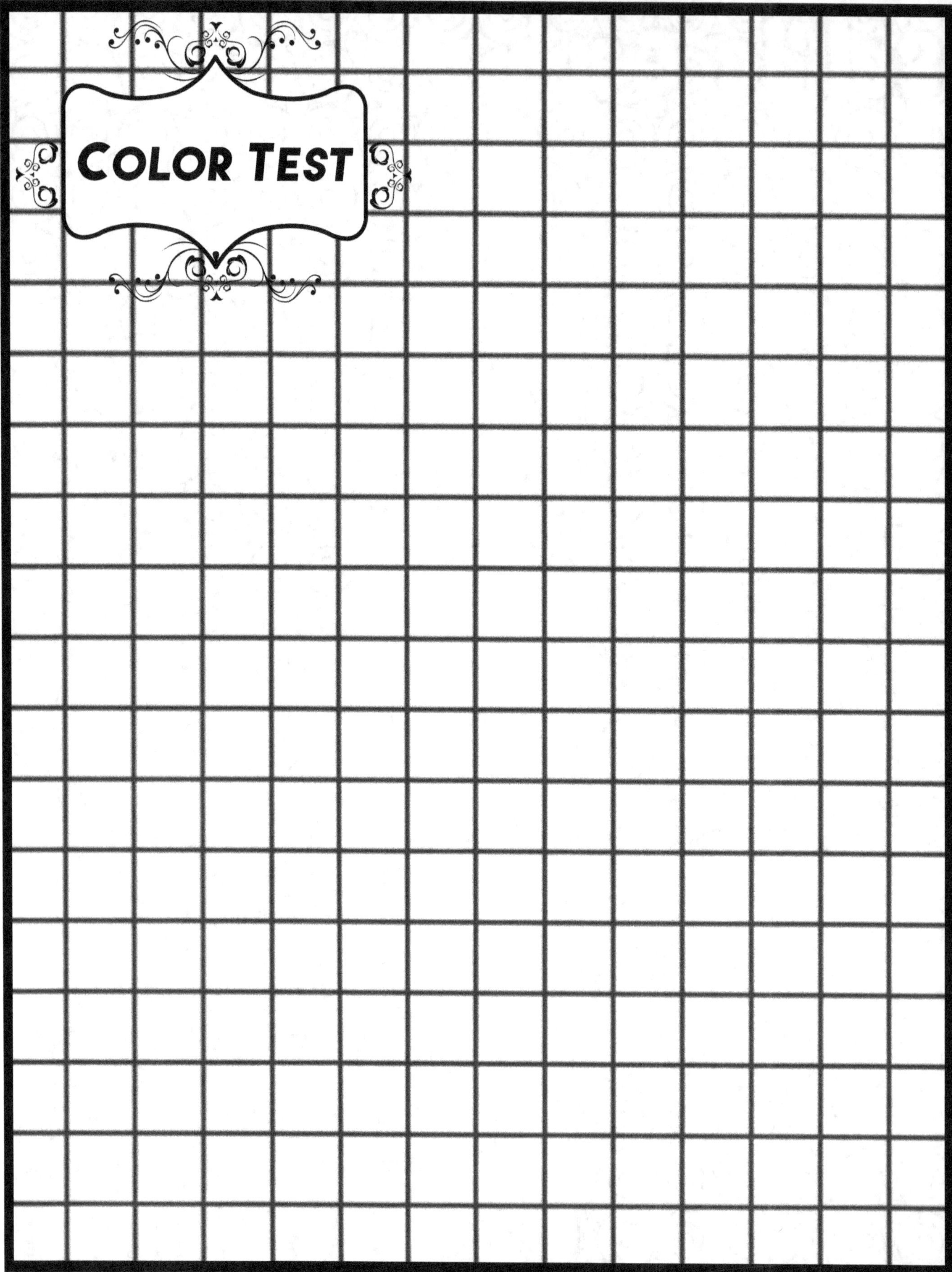

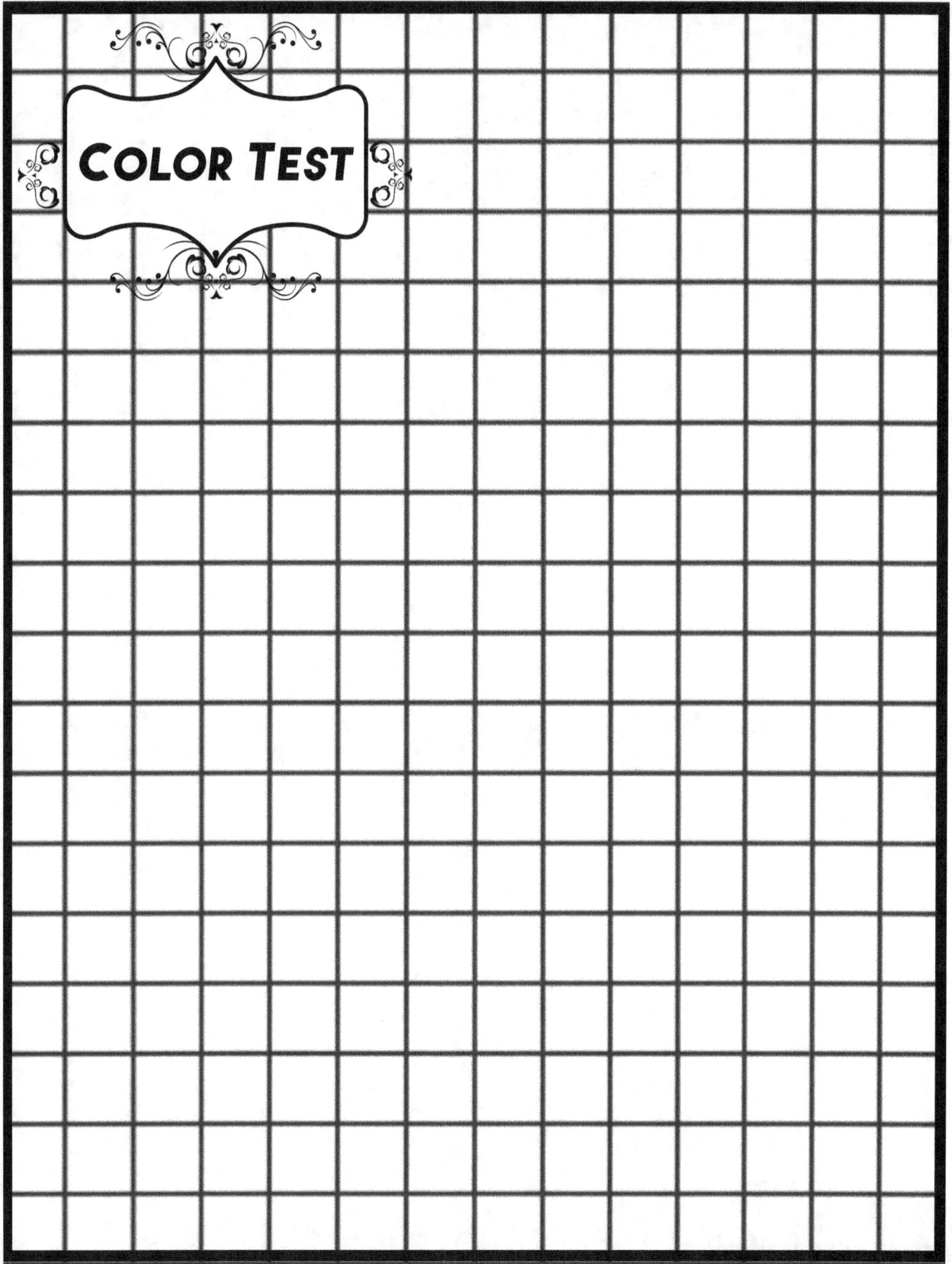
COLOR TEST